The Complete Air Fryer Breakfast Cookbook

50 Healthy and Tasty Keto Recipes for your Breakfast

Lydia Gorman

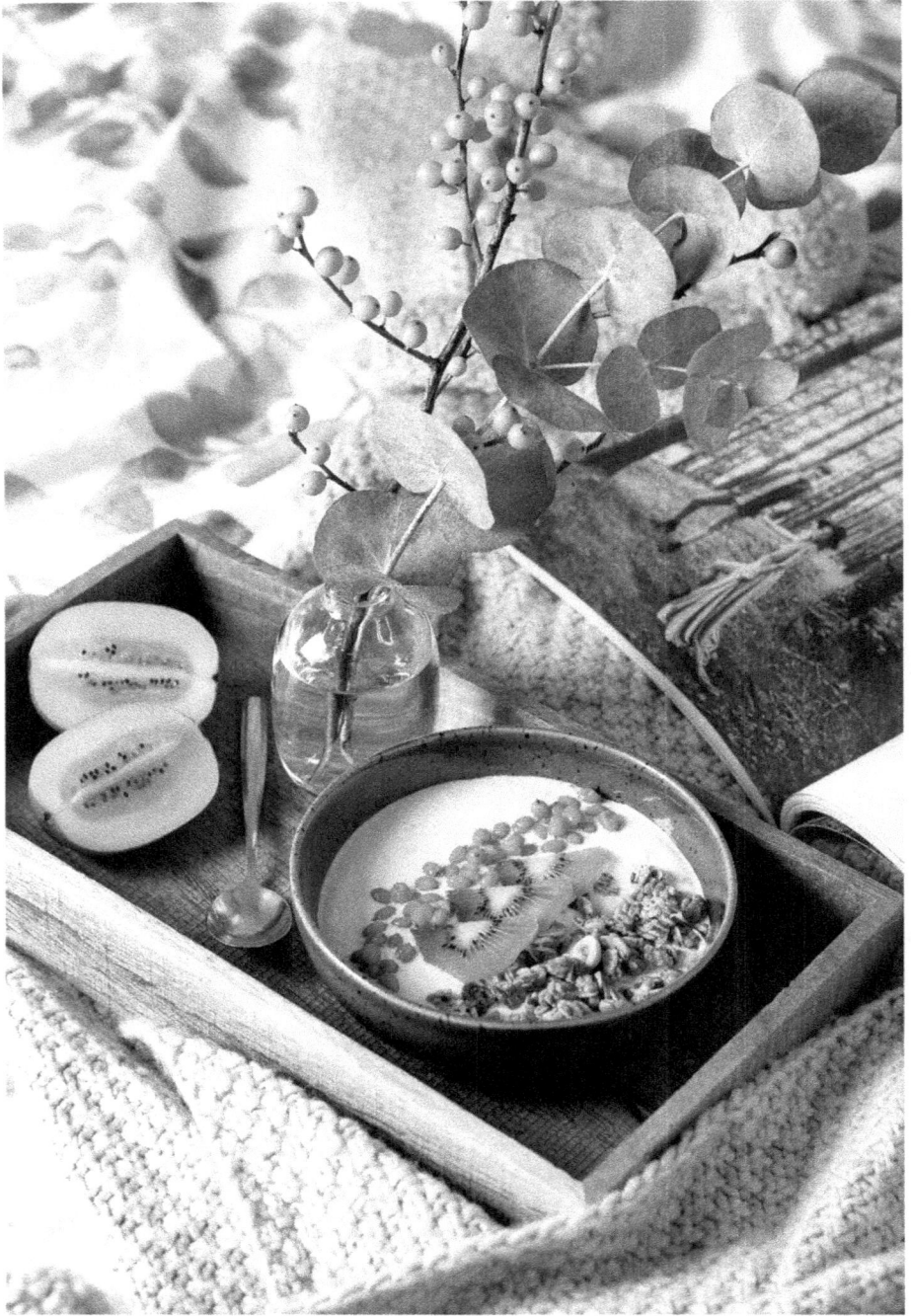

Table of Contents

Introduction

What's the difference between an air fryer and deep fryer? Air fryers bake food at a high temperature with a high-powered fan, while deep fryers cook food in a vat of oil that has been heated up to a specific temperature. Both cook food quickly, but an air fryer requires practically zero preheat time while a deep fryer can take upwards of 10 minutes. Air fryers also require little to no oil and deep fryers require a lot that absorb into the food. Food comes out crispy and juicy in both appliances, but don't taste the same, usually because deep fried foods are coated in batter that cook differently in an air fryer vs a deep fryer. Battered foods needs to be sprayed with oil before cooking in an air fryer to help them color and get crispy, while the hot oil soaks into the batter in a deep fryer. Flour-based batters and wet batters don't cook well in an air fryer, but they come out very well in a deep fryer.

The ketogenic diet is one such example. The diet calls for a very small number of carbs to be eaten. This means food such as rice, pasta, and other starchy vegetables like potatoes are off the menu. Even relaxed versions of the keto diet minimize carbs to a large extent and this compromises the goals of many dieters. They end up having to exert large amounts of willpower to follow the diet. This doesn't do them any favors since willpower is like a muscle. At some point, it tires and this is when the dieter goes right back to their old pattern of eating. I have personal experience with this. In terms of health benefits, the keto diet offers the most. The reduction of carbs forces your body to mobilize fat and this results in automatic fat loss and better health.

Feel free to mix and match the recipes you see in here and play around with them. Eating is supposed to be fun! Unfortunately, we've associated fun eating with unhealthy food. This doesn't have to be the case. The air fryer, combined with the Mediterranean diet, will make your mealtimes fun-filled again and full of taste. There's no grease and messy cleanups to deal with anymore. Are you excited yet?

You should be! You're about to embark on a journey full of air fried goodness!

Coconut & Oat Cookies

Prep + Cook Time: 30 minutes

4 Servings

INGREDIENTS

¾ cup flour

4 tbsp sugar

½ cup oats

1 egg

¼ cup coconut flakes

Filling:

1 tbsp white chocolate melted

4 tbsp butter

½ cup powdered sugar

1 tsp vanilla extract

DIRECTIONS

In a bowl, beat egg, sugar, oats, and coconut flakes with an electric mixer.

Fold in the flour.

Drop spoonfuls of the batter onto a greased baking sheet and cook in the air fryer at 350 F for 18 minutes on Bake.

Let cool to firm up and resemble cookies.

Cook in batches if needed.

Meanwhile, prepare the filling by beating all ingredients together.

Spread the filling on half of the cookies.

Top with the other halves to make cookie sandwiches.

Paprika Rarebit

Prep + Cook Time: 15 minutes

2 Servings

INGREDIENTS

4 slices bread toasted

1 tsp smoked paprika

2 eggs beaten

1 tsp dijon mustard

4 ½ oz cheddar cheese grated

Salt and black pepper to taste

DIRECTIONS

In a bowl, combine the eggs, mustard, cheddar cheese, and paprika.

Season with salt and pepper.

Spread the mixture on the toasts.

AirFry the slices in the preheated air fryer for 10 minutes at 360 F.

Quick Feta Triangles

Prep + Cook Time: 30 minutes

3 Servings

INGREDIENTS

1 cup feta cheese 1 onion, chopped

2 tbsp parsley, chopped

1 egg yolk

2 tbsp olive oil

3 sheets filo pastry

DIRECTIONS

Cut each of the filo sheets into 3 equal-sized strips.

Brush the strips with some olive oil.

In a bowl, mix onion, feta, egg yolk, and parsley.

Divide the mixture between the strips and fold each diagonally to make triangles.

Arrange them on a greased baking pan and brush the tops with the remaining olive oil.

Place in the fryer and Bake for 8 minutes at 360 F.

Serve warm.

Turkey Sausage

Preparation Time: 10 minutes

Cooking Time: 10 minutes

Serve: 8

Ingredients:

2lbs ground turkey

1 tsp dried thyme

1 tsp paprika

2 tsp garlic powder

2 tsp dry sage

2 tsp fennel seeds

1 tsp sea salt

Directions:

Add ground meat and remaining ingredients into the mixing bowl and mix until well combined.

Take 2-3 tablespoon of meat mixture and flatten into patties.

Place the cooking tray in the air fryer basket.

Select Air Fry mode. Set time to 10 minutes and temperature 370 F then press START.

The air fryer display will prompt you to ADD FOOD once the temperature is reached then place sausage patties in the air fryer basket.

Serve and enjoy.

Savory Breakfast Casserole

Preparation Time: 10 minutes

Cooking Time: 45 minutes

 Serve: 8

Ingredients:

12 eggs

1 tbsp hot sauce

3/4 cup heavy whipping cream

2 cups cheddar cheese, shredded

12 oz breakfast sausage

Pepper

Salt

Directions:

Heat large pan over medium-high heat.

Add sausage in a pan and cook for 5-7 minutes or until meat is no longer pink.

Add cooked sausage in a 9*13-inch baking dish.

In a large bowl, whisk eggs with hot sauce, cream, cheese, pepper, and salt.

Pour egg mixture over sausage in baking dish.

Cover dish with foil.

Select Bake mode.

Set time to 40 minutes and temperature 350 F then press START.

The air fryer display will prompt you to ADD FOOD once the temperature is reached then place the baking dish in the air fryer basket.

Serve and enjoy.

Zucchini Spinach Egg Casserole

Preparation Time: 10 minutes

Cooking Time: 30 minutes

Serve: 8

Ingredients:

10 eggs

1/4 cup goat cheese, crumbled

4 cherry tomatoes, cut in half

1/3 cup cheddar cheese, grated

1/3 cup ham, chopped

1 small zucchini, sliced

1/2 cup spinach

2/3 cup heavy cream

Pepper

Salt

Directions:

In a bowl, whisk eggs with cream, pepper, and salt.

Stir in cheddar cheese, ham, zucchini, and spinach.

Pour egg mixture into the greased baking dish.

Top with goat cheese and cherry tomatoes.

Cover dish with foil.

Select Bake mode.

Set time to 30 minutes and temperature 350 F then press START.

The air fryer display will prompt you to ADD FOOD once the temperature is reached then place the baking dish in the air fryer basket.

Serve and enjoy.

Ham Cheese Casserole

Preparation Time: 10 minutes

Cooking Time: 35 minutes

Serve: 12

Ingredients:

12 eggs

1/2 cup cheddar cheese, shredded

4 oz cream cheese, cubed

2 cups ham, diced

1 cup heavy cream

1/4 tsp pepper

1/4 tsp salt

Directions:

In a large bowl, whisk eggs with cream, pepper, and salt.

Stir in cheddar cheese, cream cheese, and ham.

Pour egg mixture into the greased 9*13-inch baking dish.

Cover dish with foil.

Select Bake mode.

Set time to 35 minutes and temperature 350 F then press START.

The air fryer display will prompt you to ADD FOOD once the temperature is reached then place the baking dish in the air fryer basket.

Serve and enjoy.

Crustless Cheese Egg Quiche

Preparation Time: 10 minutes

Cooking Time: 45 minutes

Serve: 6

Ingredients:

12 eggs

12 tbsp butter, melted

4 oz cream cheese, softened

8 oz cheddar cheese, grated

Pepper

Salt

Directions:

In a bowl, whisk eggs with butter, cream cheese, half cheddar cheese, pepper, and salt.

Pour egg mixture into the greased 9.5-inch pie pan.

Sprinkle remaining cheese on top.

Cover dish with foil.

Select Bake mode.

Set time to 45 minutes and temperature 325 F then press START.

The air fryer display will prompt you to ADD FOOD once the temperature is reached then place the pie pan in the air fryer basket. Serve and enjoy.

Veggie Egg Casserole

Preparation Time: 10 minutes

Cooking Time: 30 minutes

Serve: 10

Ingredients:

12 eggs, lightly beaten

1 cup cheddar cheese, shredded

2 bell pepper, diced

1 tsp garlic, minced

1 cup onion, chopped

5 bacon slices, cooked and chopped

1 tbsp olive oil

1/4 tsp pepper

1/2 tsp sea salt

Directions:

Heat oil in a pan over medium heat.

Add garlic and onion in a pan and sauté until onion is softened.

In a bowl, whisk eggs with pepper and salt.

Stir in cheddar cheese, bell pepper, bacon, garlic, and onion.

Pour egg mixture into the greased 9*13-inch baking dish.

Cover dish with foil.

Select Bake mode.

Set time to 30 minutes and temperature 350 F then press START.

The air fryer display will prompt you to ADD FOOD once the temperature is reached then place the baking dish in the air fryer basket.

Serve and enjoy.

Cauliflower Muffins

Preparation Time: 10 minutes

Cooking Time: 25 minutes

Serve: 12

Ingredients:

5 eggs

1 cup cheddar cheese, shredded

1/2 tsp garlic powder

1/2 cup onion, chopped

1/2 cup baby spinach

6 oz ham, diced

3 cups cauliflower rice, squeeze out excess liquid

Pepper

Salt

Directions:

In a bowl, whisk eggs with cheese, garlic powder, pepper, and salt.

Stir in onion, spinach, ham, and cauliflower rice.

Pour egg mixture into the silicone muffin molds.

Select Bake mode.

Set time to 25 minutes and temperature 375 F then press START.

The air fryer display will prompt you to ADD FOOD once the temperature is reached then place muffin molds in the air fryer basket.

Serve and enjoy.

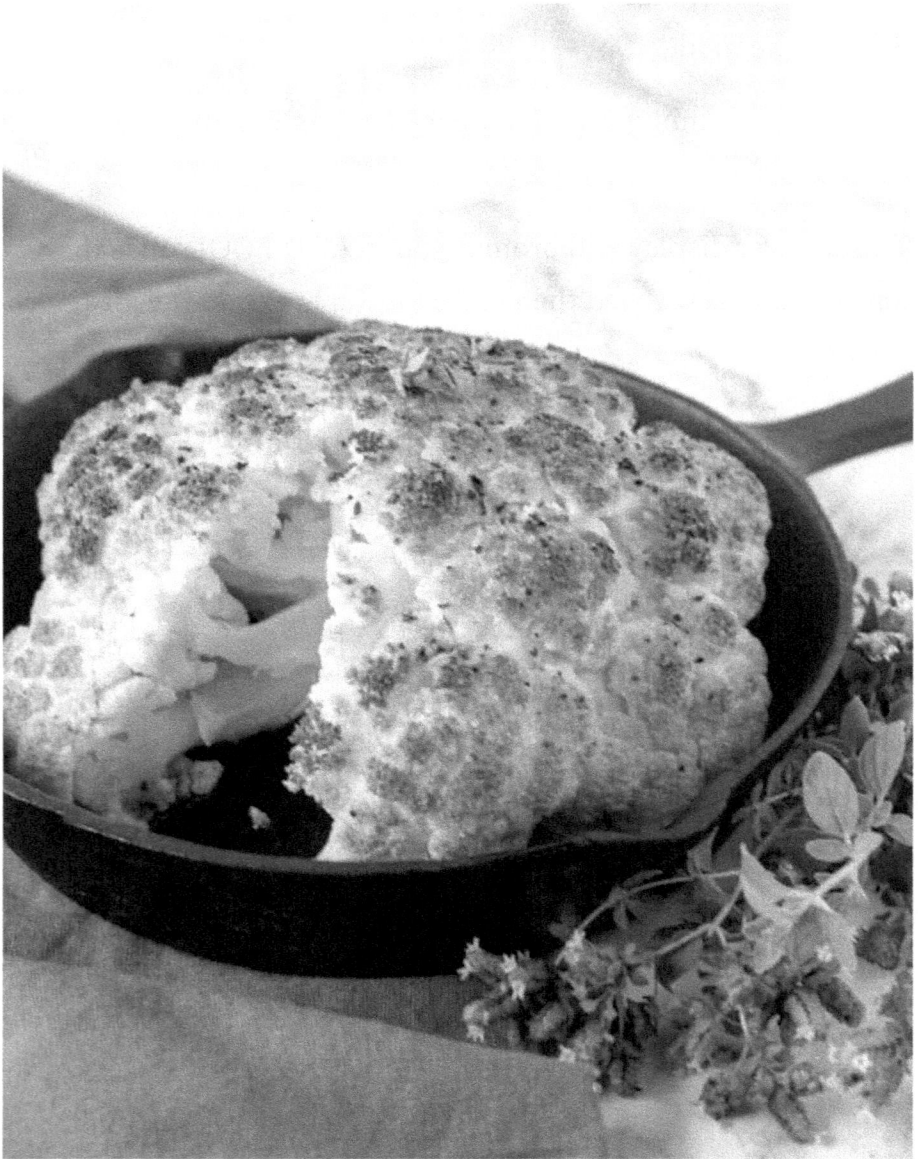

Delicious Zucchini Frittata

Preparation Time: 10 minutes

Cooking Time: 30 minutes

Serve: 4

Ingredients:

8 eggs

1 tbsp parsley, chopped

3 tbsp parmesan cheese, grated

2 small zucchinis, grated

1/2 cup pancetta, chopped

2 tbsp olive oil

Pepper

Salt

Directions:

Heat oil in a pan over medium heat.

Add zucchini and pancetta into the pan and sauté for 8-10 minutes.

In a bowl, whisk eggs with parsley, cheese, pepper, and salt.

Stir in sauteed zucchini and pancetta.

Pour egg mixture into the greased 8-inch baking dish.

Select Bake mode.

Set time to 20 minutes and temperature 350 F then press START.

The air fryer display will prompt you to ADD FOOD once the temperature is reached then place the baking dish in the air fryer basket.

Serve and enjoy.

Cheesy Zucchini Quiche

Preparation Time: 10 minutes

Cooking Time: 60 minutes

Serve: 8

Ingredients:

6 eggs

2 medium zucchinis, shredded & Squeeze out excess liquid

2 tbsp fresh parsley, chopped

1/2 cup olive oil

 1 cup cheddar cheese, shredded

1 cup almond flour

1/2 tsp dried basil

 2 garlic cloves, minced

1 tbsp dry onion, minced

2 tbsp parmesan cheese, grated

1/2 tsp salt

Directions:

Add all ingredients into the large bowl and mix until well combined.

Pour mixture into the greased 9-inch pie dish.

Cover pie dish with foil.

Select Bake mode.

Set time to 60 minutes and temperature 350 F then press START.

The air fryer display will prompt you to ADD FOOD once the temperature is reached then place the pie dish in the air fryer basket.

Slice and serve.

Tomato Kale Egg Muffins

Preparation Time: 10 minutes

Cooking Time: 25 minutes

Serve: 6

Ingredients:

5 eggs 3 tomatoes, chopped

2/3 cup unsweetened almond milk

1 green onion, chopped

1/2 cup kale, shredded

1/8 tsp pepper

1/4 tsp salt

Directions:

In a bowl, whisk eggs with milk, pepper, and salt.

Stir in tomatoes, kale, and onion.

Pour egg mixture into the silicone muffin molds.

Select Bake mode.

Set time to 25 minutes and temperature 350 F then press START.

The air fryer display will prompt you to ADD FOOD once the temperature is reached then place muffin molds in the air fryer basket.

Serve and enjoy.

Healthy Breakfast Donuts

Preparation Time: 10 minutes

Cooking Time: 20 minutes

Serve: 6

Ingredients:

4 eggs

1/2 tsp instant coffee

1/3 cup unsweetened almond milk

1 tbsp liquid stevia

3 tbsp cocoa powder

1/4 cup butter, melted

1/3 cup coconut flour

1/2 tsp baking soda

1/2 tsp baking powder

Directions:

Add all ingredients into the large bowl and mix until well combined.

Pour batter into the silicone donut molds.

Select Bake mode.

Set time to 20 minutes and temperature 350 F then press START.

The air fryer display will prompt you to ADD FOOD once the temperature is reached then place donut molds in the air fryer basket.

Serve and enjoy.

Simple & Easy Breakfast Quiche

Preparation Time: 10 minutes

Cooking Time: 45 minutes

Serve: 6

Ingredients:

6 eggs

1 cup unsweetened almond milk

1 cup tomatoes, chopped

1 cup cheddar cheese, grated

1 tsp garlic powder

Pepper

Salt

Directions:

In a bowl, whisk eggs with cheese, milk, garlic powder, pepper, and salt.

Stir in tomatoes.

Pour egg mixture into the greased pie dish.

Cover dish with foil. Select Bake mode.

Set time to 45 minutes and temperature 350 F then press START.

The air fryer display will prompt you to ADD FOOD once the temperature is reached then place the pie dish in the air fryer basket.

Serve and enjoy.

Parmesan Zucchini Frittata

Preparation Time: 10 minutes

 Cooking Time: 30 minutes

Serve: 4

Ingredients:

8 eggs

2 zucchinis, chopped and cooked

1 tbsp fresh parsley, chopped

3 tbsp parmesan cheese, grated

1 tsp garlic powder

Pepper

Salt

Directions:

In a large bowl, whisk eggs with garlic powder, pepper, and salt.

Stir in parsley, cheese, and zucchini.

Pour egg mixture into the greased baking dish.

Cover dish with foil.

Select Bake mode.

Set time to 30 minutes and temperature 350 F then press START.

The air fryer display will prompt you to ADD FOOD once the temperature is reached then place the baking dish in the air fryer basket.

Serve and enjoy

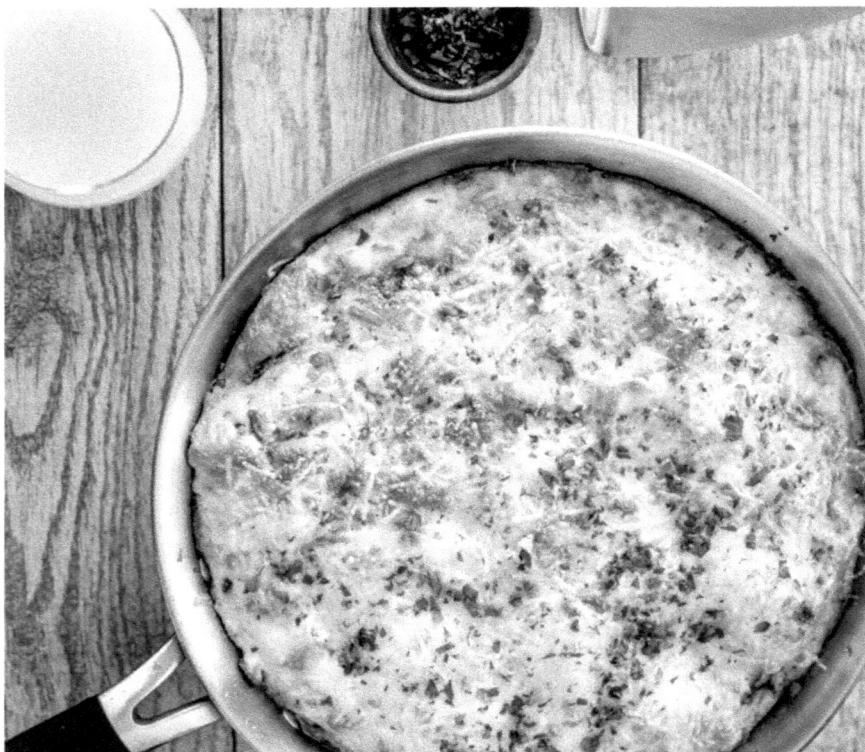

Bake Cheese Omelet

Preparation Time: 10 minutes

Cooking Time: 25 minutes

Serve: 6

Ingredients:

8 eggs

1/4 cup cheddar cheese, shredded

2 tbsp green onions, chopped

1/4 tsp garlic powder

1/2 cup unsweetened almond milk

1/2 cup half and half

Pepper

Salt

Directions:

In a bowl, whisk eggs with milk, half and half, garlic powder, pepper, and salt.

Stir in green onion and cheese.

Pour egg mixture into the greased 8-inch baking dish.

Cover dish with foil.

Select Bake mode.

Set time to 25 minutes and temperature 350 F then press START.

The air fryer display will prompt you to ADD FOOD once the temperature is reached then place the baking dish in the air fryer basket.

Serve and enjoy.

Sun-dried Tomatoes Egg Cups

Preparation Time: 10 minutes

Cooking Time: 20 minutes

Serve: 12

Ingredients:

6 eggs

1 1/2 tbsp basil, chopped

2 tsp olive oil

1/2 cup feta cheese, crumbled

4 cherry tomatoes, chopped

4 sun- dried tomatoes, chopped

Pepper

Salt

Directions:

In a bowl, whisk eggs with pepper and salt.

Add remaining ingredients and stir well.

Pour egg mixture into the silicone muffin molds.

Select Bake mode.

Set time to 20 minutes and temperature 400 F then press START.

The air fryer display will prompt you to ADD FOOD once the temperature is reached then place muffin molds in the air fryer basket.

Serve and enjoy.

Mushroom Kale Egg Cups

Preparation Time: 10 minutes

Cooking Time: 15 minutes

Serve: 8

Ingredients:

6 eggs

1 cup mushrooms, diced

1 cup kale, chopped

1 tsp olive oil

2 tbsp onion, minced

1/2 cup Swiss cheese, shredded

Pepper

Salt

Directions:

Heat oil in a pan over medium-high heat.

Add mushrooms and sauté for 2-3 minutes.

Add onion and kale and sauté for 2 minutes.

Remove pan from heat.

In a bowl, whisk eggs with pepper and salt.

Stir in sautéed mushroom kale mixture and shredded cheese.

Pour egg mixture into the silicone muffin molds. Select Bake mode.

Set time to 15 minutes and temperature 350 F then press START.

The air fryer display will prompt you to ADD FOOD once the temperature is reached then place muffin molds in the air fryer basket.

Serve and enjoy.

Sun-dried Tomatoes Kale Egg Cups

Preparation Time: 10 minutes

Cooking Time: 35 minutes

Serve: 12

Ingredients:

10 eggs

1/4 cup sun-dried tomatoes, chopped

1 cup unsweetened coconut milk

1/4 cup sausage, sliced

1/4 cup kale, chopped

Pepper

Salt

Directions:

In a large bowl, add all ingredients and whisk until well combined.

Pour egg mixture into the silicone muffin molds.

Select Bake mode.

Set time to 35 minutes and temperature 350 F then press START.

The air fryer display will prompt you to ADD FOOD once the temperature is reached then place muffin molds in the air fryer basket.

Serve and enjoy.

Roasted Pepper Egg Cups

Preparation Time: 10 minutes

Cooking Time: 20 minutes

Serve: 12

Ingredients:

8 eggs

1 cup roasted red peppers, chopped

1/4 cup unsweetened almond milk

1 cup spinach, chopped

1/2 tsp salt

Directions:

In a bowl, whisk eggs with coconut milk and salt.

Add spinach, green onion, and red peppers to the egg mixture and stir to combine.

Pour egg mixture into the silicone muffin molds.

Select Bake mode.

Set time to 20 minutes and temperature 350 F then press START.

The air fryer display will prompt you to ADD FOOD once the temperature is reached then place muffin molds in the air fryer basket.

Serve and enjoy.

Spinach Bacon Egg Bake

Preparation Time: 10 minutes

Cooking Time: 45 minutes

Serve: 6

Ingredients:

10 eggs

3 cups baby spinach, chopped

1 tbsp olive oil

10 bacon sliced, cooked and crumbled

2 large tomatoes, sliced

1/2 tsp salt

Directions:

Heat oil in a pan over medium heat.

Add spinach and cook until spinach wilted.

In a mixing bowl, whisk eggs with salt.

Stir in spinach.

Pour egg mixture into the greased 9-inch baking dish.

Cover dish with foil.

Select Bake mode.

Set time to 45 minutes and temperature 350 F then press START.

The air fryer display will prompt you to ADD FOOD once the temperature is reached then place the baking dish in the air fryer basket.

Serve and enjoy.

Egg Casserole

Preparation Time: 10 minutes

Cooking Time: 30 minutes

Serve: 2

Ingredients:

5 eggs

2 tbsp heavy cream

3 tbsp tomato sauce

2 tbsp parmesan cheese, grated

Directions:

In a bowl, whisk eggs with cream.

Stir in cheese and tomato sauce.

Pour egg mixture into the greased baking dish.

Cover dish with foil. Select Bake mode.

Set time to 30 minutes and temperature 350 F then press START.

The air fryer display will prompt you to ADD FOOD once the temperature is reached then place the baking dish in the air fryer basket.

Serve and enjoy.

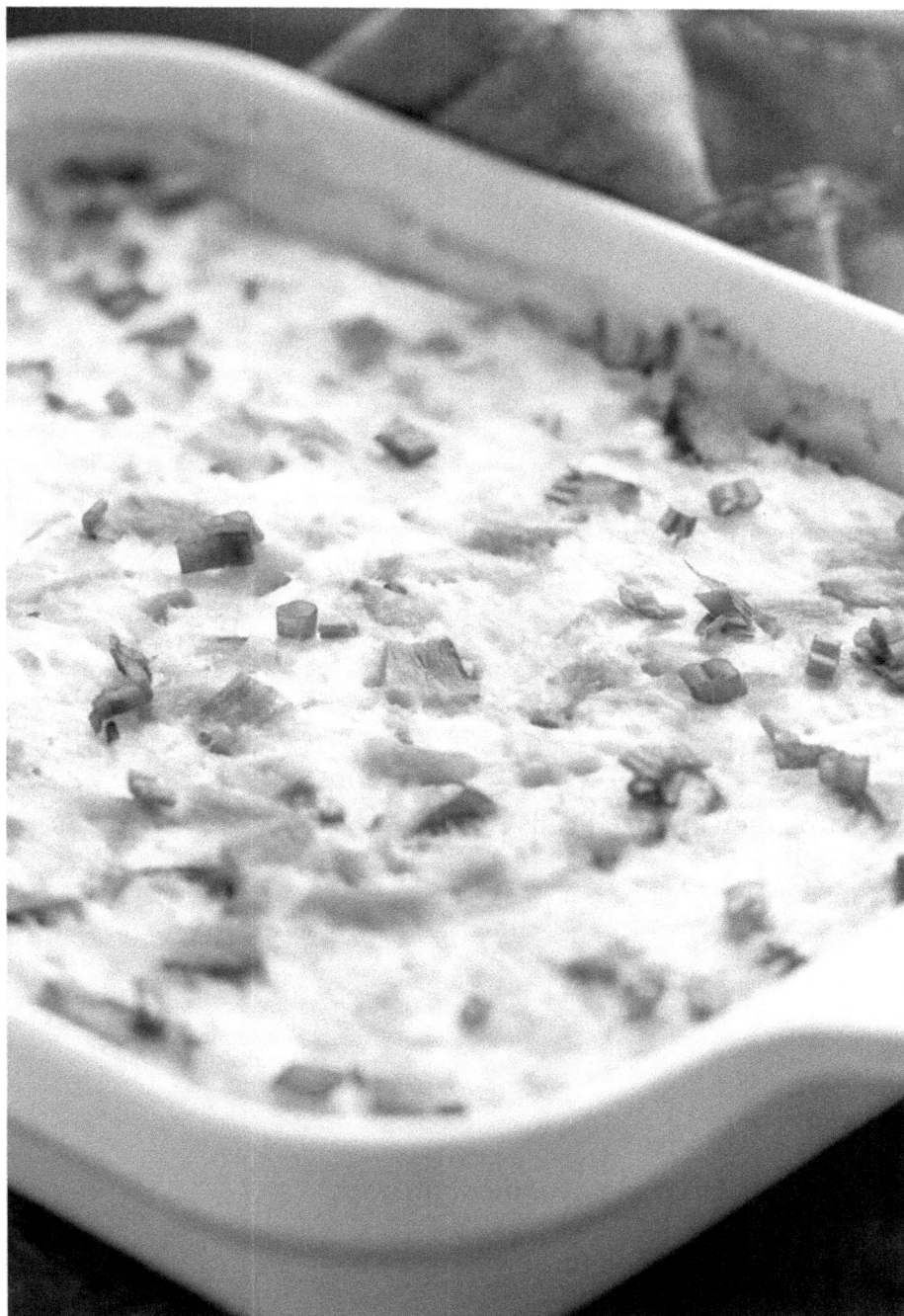

Spinach Egg Bake

Preparation Time: 10 minutes

Cooking Time: 35 minutes

Serve: 6

Ingredients:

8 eggs, beaten

1 1/2 cups mozzarella

1 tsp olive oil

5 oz fresh spinach

1 tsp spike seasoning

1/3 cup green onion, sliced

Pepper

Salt

Directions:

Heat oil in a large pan over medium heat.

Add spinach and cook until wilted.

Transfer cooked spinach into the casserole dish and spread well.

Spread onion and cheese on top.

In a bowl, whisk together eggs, pepper, spike seasoning, and salt.

Pour egg mixture over spinach mixture.

Cover dish with foil.

Select Bake mode.

Set time to 35 minutes and temperature 375 F then press START.

The air fryer display will prompt you to ADD FOOD once the temperature is reached then place a casserole dish in the air fryer basket.

Slice and serve.

Spinach Pepper Breakfast Egg Cups

Preparation Time: 10 minutes

Cooking Time: 20 minutes

Serve: 12

Ingredients:

9 eggs 1 cup bell peppers, chopped

1/2 cup onion, sliced

1 tbsp olive oil

8 oz ground sausage

1/4 cup unsweetened almond milk

1/2 tsp oregano

1 1/2 cups spinach

Pepper

Salt

Directions:

Add ground sausage in a pan and sauté over medium heat until browned.

Add olive oil, oregano, bell pepper, and onion and sauté until onion is translucent.

Add spinach and cook until spinach is wilted.

Remove pan from heat and set aside.

In a bowl, whisk eggs, milk, pepper, and salt.

Add sausage and vegetable mixture into the egg mixture and mix well.

Pour egg mixture into the silicone muffin molds.

Select Bake mode.

Set time to 20 minutes and temperature 350 F then press START.

The air fryer display will prompt you to ADD FOOD once the temperature is reached then place muffin molds in the air fryer basket.

Serve and enjoy.

Cheddar Cheese Ham Quiche

Preparation Time: 10 minutes

Cooking Time: 40 minutes

Serve: 6

Ingredients:

8 eggs

1 cup zucchini, shredded and squeezed

1 cup ham, cooked and diced

1/2 tsp dry mustard

1/2 cup heavy cream

1 cup cheddar cheese, shredded

Pepper

Salt

Directions:

Add ham, cheddar cheese, and zucchini in a 9-inch pie dish.

In a bowl, whisk together eggs, heavy cream, and seasoning.

Pour egg mixture over ham mixture.

Cover dish with foil.

Select Bake mode.

Set time to 40 minutes and temperature 375 F then press START.

The air fryer display will prompt you to ADD FOOD once the temperature is reached then add food in the air fryer basket.

Serve and enjoy.

Coconut Jalapeno Muffins

Preparation Time: 10 minutes

Cooking Time: 20 minutes

Serve: 8

Ingredients:

5 eggs

3 tbsp jalapenos, sliced

3 tbsp erythritol

2/3 cup coconut flour

1/4 cup unsweetened coconut milk

1/3 cup coconut oil, melted

2 tsp baking powder

3/4 tsp sea salt

Directions:

In a large bowl, stir together coconut flour, baking powder, sweetener, and sea salt.

Stir in eggs, jalapenos, milk, and coconut oil until well combined.

Pour batter into the silicone muffin molds.

Select Bake mode.

Set time to 20 minutes and temperature 350 F then press START.

The air fryer display will prompt you to ADD FOOD once the temperature is reached then place muffin molds in the air fryer basket.

Serve and enjoy.

Breakfast Vegetable Quiche

Preparation Time: 10 minutes

 Cooking Time: 40 minutes

Serve: 6

Ingredients:

8 egg whites

1 cup gruyere cheese, shredded

1/4 cup onion, diced

2 cups spinach, steamed & squeeze out excess liquid

4 pieces roasted red peppers, sliced

1/2 cup cherry tomatoes, halved

1 garlic cloves, minced

1/2 cup unsweetened coconut milk

Pepper

Salt

Directions:

Spray pan with cooking spray and heat over medium-high heat.

Add garlic and onion and sauté until softened.

In a bowl, whisk egg whites, cheese, and milk.

Add sautéed onion and garlic into the egg mixture and stir well.

Layer tomatoes, roasted peppers, and spinach in a greased baking dish.

Pour egg mixture over the vegetables.

Cover dish with foil.

Select Bake mode.

Set time to 40 minutes and temperature 350 F then press START.

The air fryer display will prompt you to ADD FOOD once the temperature is reached then place the baking dish in the air fryer basket.

Serve and enjoy.

Mediterranean Avocado Toast

Prep + Cook Time: 7 minutes

2 Serving

INGREDIENTS

2 slices thick whole grain bread

4 thin tomato slices

1 ripe avocado, pitted, peeled, and sliced

1 tbsp olive oil

1 tbsp pinch of salt

½ tsp chili flakes

DIRECTIONS

Preheat air fryer to 370 F.

Arrange the bread slices on the fryer and toast on Bake mode.

Add the avocado to a bowl and mash it up with a fork until smooth.

Season with salt.

When the toasted bread is ready, remove it to a plate.

Drizzle with olive oil and arrange the thin tomato slices on top.

Spread the avocado mash on top.

Sprinkle the toasts with chili flakes and serve

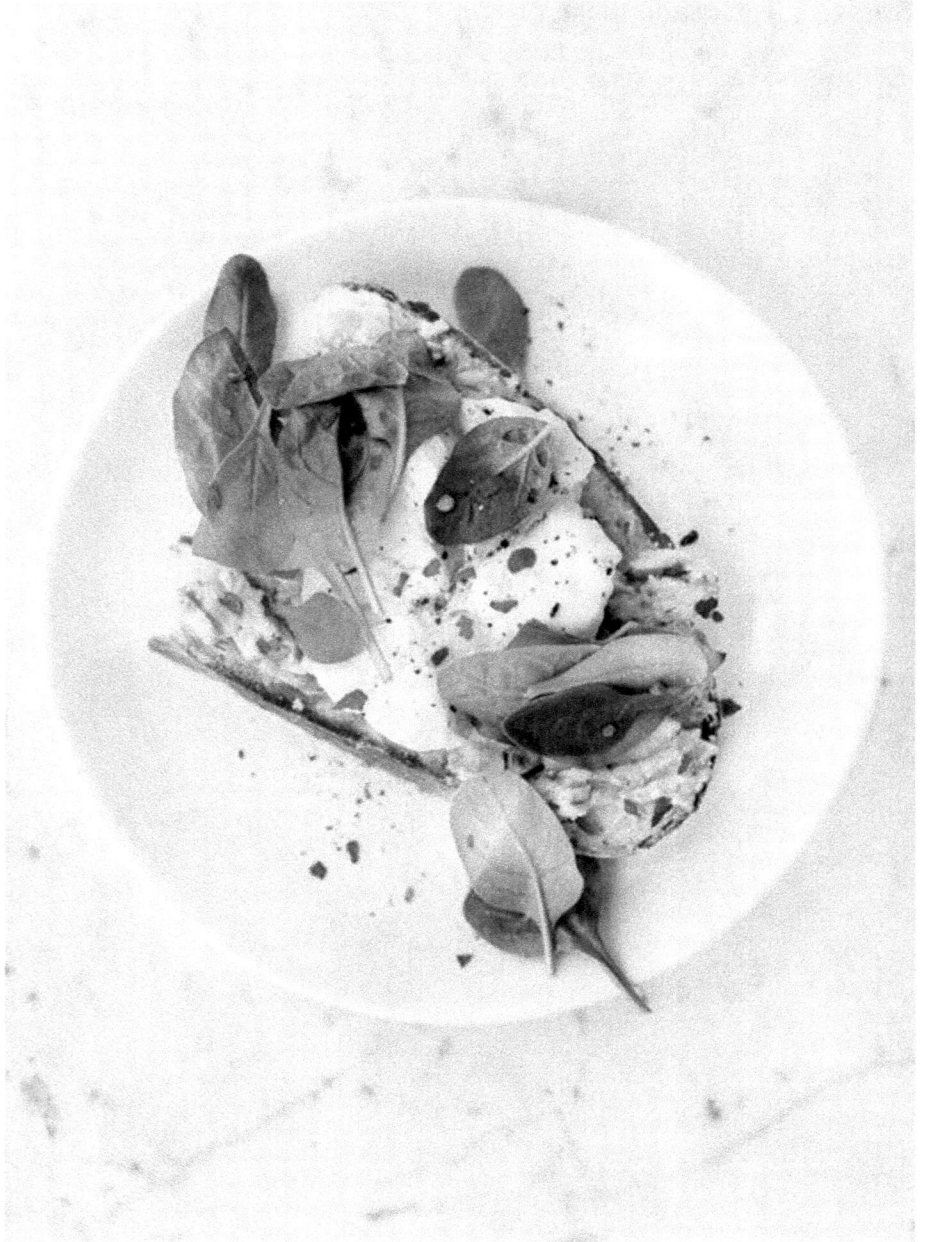

Bacon & Egg Sandwich

Prep + Cook Time: 10 minutes

1 Serving

INGREDIENTS

1 egg, fried

1 slice English bacon

Salt and black pepper to taste

2 bread slices

½ tbsp butter, softened

DIRECTIONS

Preheat air fryer to 400 F.

Spread butter on one side of the bread slices.

Add the fried egg on top and season with salt and black pepper.

Top with bacon and cover with the other slice of bread.

Place in the fryer's cooking basket and AirFry for 4-6 minutes.

Serve warm.

Grilled Apple & Brie Sandwich

Prep + Cook Time: 10 minutes

1 Serving

INGREDIENTS

2 bread slices

½ apple, thinly sliced

2 tsp butter

2 oz brie cheese, thinly sliced

DIRECTIONS

Spread butter on the outside of the bread slices and top with apple slices.

Place brie slices on top of the apple and cover with the other slice of bread.

Bake in the fryer for 5 minutes at 350 F.

When ready, remove and cut diagonally to serve.

Air Fried Sourdough Sandwiches

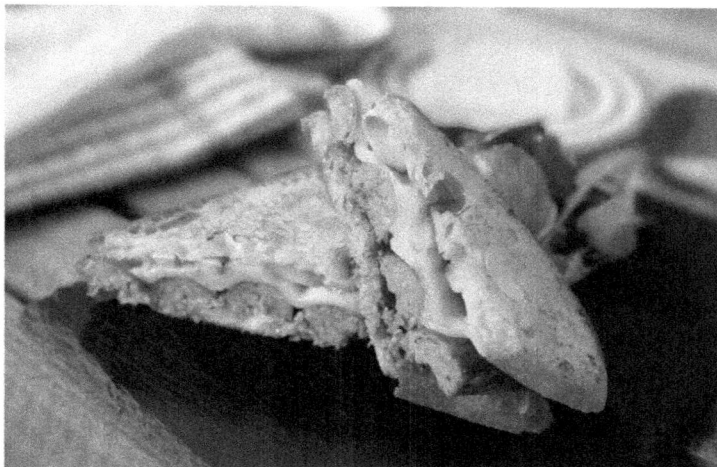

Prep + Cook Time: 20 minutes

2 Servings

INGREDIENTS

4 slices sourdough bread

2 tbsp mayonnaise

2 slices ham

2 lettuce leaves

1 tomato, sliced

2 slices mozzarella cheese

DIRECTIONS

Preheat air fryer to 350 F.

On a clean working board, lay the bread slices and spread them with mayonnaise.

Top 2 of the slices with ham, lettuce leaves, tomato slices, and mozzarella.

Cover with the remaining bread slices to form two sandwiches.

AirFry for 12 minutes, flipping once. Serve hot.

Sausage & Egg Casserole

Prep + Cook Time: 20 minutes

6 Servings

INGREDIENTS

1 lb ground sausages

6 eggs

1 red pepper, diced

1 green pepper, diced

1 yellow pepper, diced

1 sweet onion, diced

1 cup cheddar cheese, shredded

Salt and black pepper to taste

2 tbsp fresh parsley, chopped

DIRECTIONS

Place a skillet over medium heat on a stovetop.

Add the sausages and cook until brown, turning occasionally, about 5 minutes.

Once done, drain any excess fat derived from cooking and set aside.

Arrange the sausages on the bottom of a greased casserole dish that fits in your air fryer.

Top with onion, red pepper, green pepper, and yellow pepper.

Sprinkle the cheese on top.

In a bowl, beat the eggs with salt and pepper.

Pour the mixture over the cheese.

Place the casserole dish in the air fryer basket and bake at 360 F for 15 minutes.

Serve warm garnished with fresh parsley.

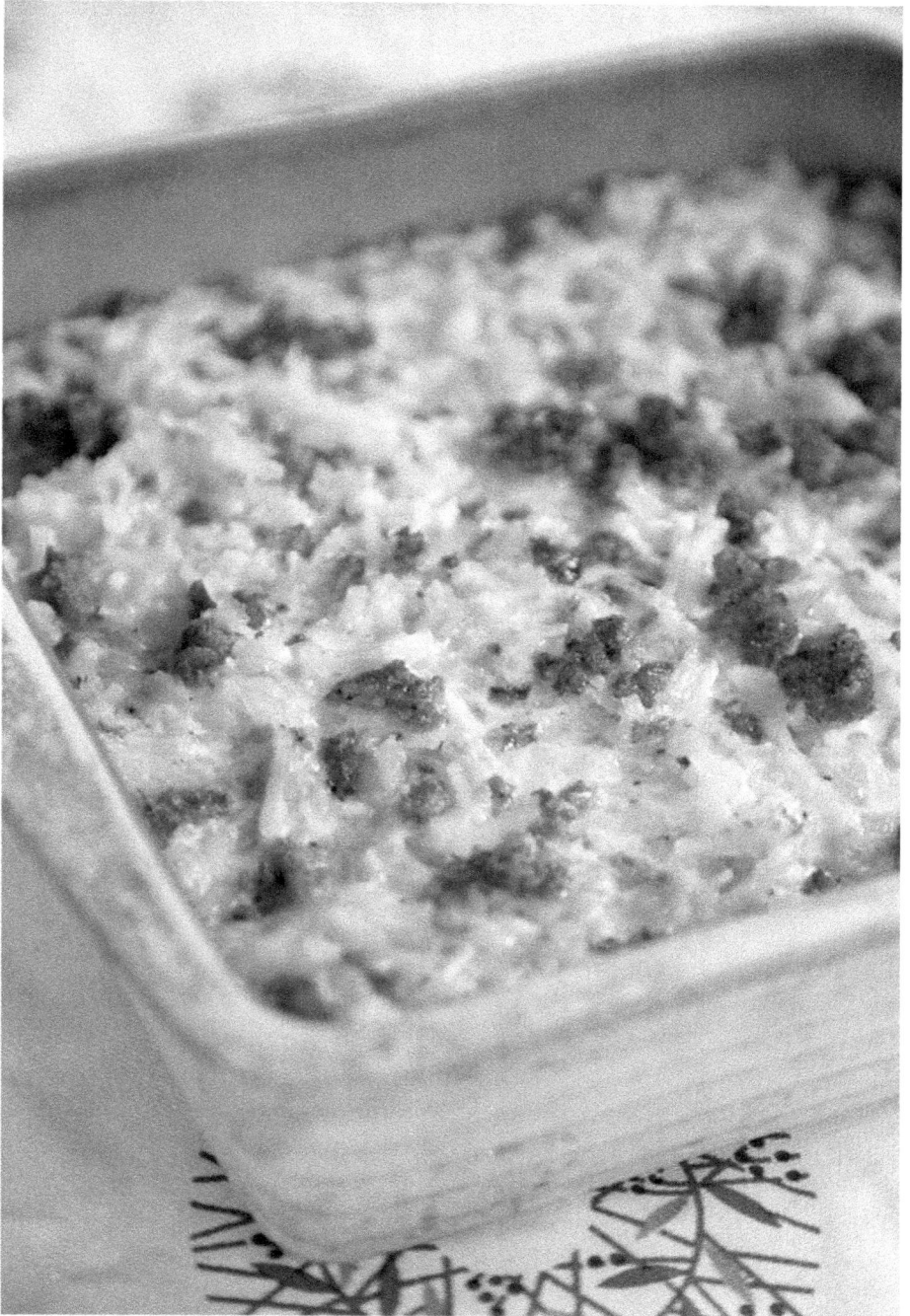

Cheese & Ham Breakfast Egg Cups

Prep + Cook Time: 20 minutes

6 Servings

INGREDIENTS

4 eggs, beaten

1 tbsp olive oil

½ cup Colby cheese, shredded

2 ¼ cups frozen hash browns, thawed

1 cup smoked ham, chopped

½ tsp Cajun seasoning

DIRECTIONS

Preheat air fryer to 360 F.

Gather 12 silicone muffin cups and coat with olive oil.

Whisk the eggs, hash browns, smoked ham, Colby cheese, and Cajun seasoning in a medium bowl and add a heaping spoonful into each muffin cup.

Put the muffin cups in the fryer basket and AirFry 8-10 minutes until golden brown and the center is set.

Transfer to a wire rack to cool completely.

Serve.

Prosciutto & Mozzarella Bruschetta

Prep + Cook Time: 7 minutes

2 Servings

INGREDIENTS

½ cup tomatoes, finely chopped

3 oz mozzarella cheese, grated

3 prosciutto slices, chopped

1 tbsp olive oil

1 tsp dried basil

6 small French bread slices

DIRECTIONS

Preheat air fryer to 350 F.

Add in the bread slices and toast for 3 minutes on AirFry mode.

Remove and top the bread with tomatoes, prosciutto, and mozzarella cheese.

Sprinkle basil all over and drizzle with olive oil.

Return to the fryer and cook for 1 more minute, just to heat through.

Serve warm.

Mushroom & Chicken Mini Pizzas

Prep + Cook Time: 15 minutes

1 Serving

INGREDIENTS

½ cup chicken meat, thinly chopped

¼ cup tomato-basil sauce

1 cup button mushrooms, sliced

1 tsp Parmesan cheese, grated

1 tsp black pepper

½ tsp garlic powder

DIRECTIONS

Preheat air fryer to 400 F.

Line a baking dish with parchment paper.

In a bowl, combine chicken with garlic and pepper.

Place spoonfuls of the chicken into the dish and flatten into rounds.

AirFryfor 8-10 minutes, remove, turn, and top with tomato-basil sauce, mushrooms, and Parmesan cheese.

Slide in the fryer and continue cooking for 5-6 minutes more until golden.

Serve.

Soppressata Pizza

Prep + Cook Time: 15 minutes

2 Servings

INGREDIENTS

1 pizza crust

½ tsp dried oregano

½ cup passata

½ cup mozzarella cheese, shredded

 4 oz soppressata, chopped

4 basil leaves

DIRECTIONS

Preheat air fryer to 370 F.

Spread the passata over the pizza crust, sprinkle with oregano, mozzarella cheese, and finish with soppressata.

Bake in the fryer for 10 minutes.

Top with basil leaves to serve.

Sausage Frittata with Parmesan

Prep + Cook Time: 15 minutes

2 Servings

INGREDIENTS

1 sausage, chopped

Salt and black pepper to taste

1 tbsp parsley, chopped

4 eggs

1 tbsp olive oil

4 cherry tomatoes, halved

2 tbsp Parmesan cheese, shredded

DIRECTIONS

Preheat air fryer to 360 F.

Place tomatoes and sausages in the air fryer's basket and cook for 5 minutes.

Remove them to a bowl and mix in eggs, salt, parsley, Parmesan cheese, olive oil, and black pepper.

Add the mixture to a greased baking pan and fit in the fryer.

Bake for 8 minutes.

Serve hot.

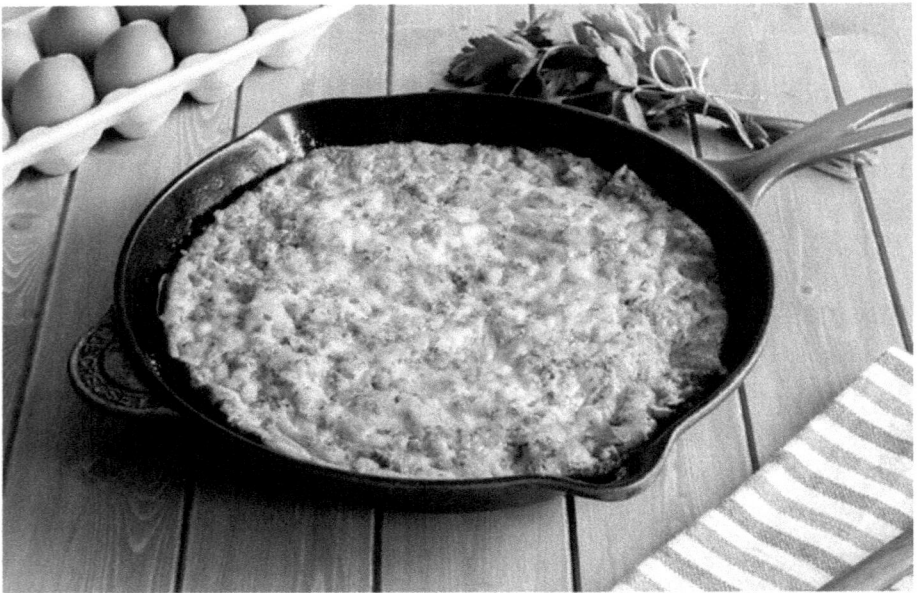

Crustless Broccoli & Mushroom Quiche

Prep + Cook Time: 25 minutes

4 Servings

INGREDIENTS

4 eggs, beaten

1 cup mushrooms, sliced

1 cup broccoli florets, steamed

½ cup cheddar cheese, shredded

½ cup mozzarella cheese, shredded

2 tbsp olive oil

¼ tsp ground allspice

Salt and black pepper to taste

DIRECTIONS

Preheat air fryer to 360 F.

Warm the olive oil in a pan over medium heat.

Sauté the mushrooms for 3-4 minutes or until soft.

Stir the broccoli for 1 minute; set aside.

Put the eggs, cheddar cheese, mozzarella cheese, allspice, salt, and pepper in a medium bowl and whisk well.

Pour the mushroom/broccoli concoction into the egg mixture and gently fold it in.

Transfer the batter to a greased baking pan.

Air fry for 5 minutes, then stir the mixture and air fry until the eggs are done, about 3-5 more minutes.

Cut into wedges and serve.

Zucchini Muffins

Prep + Cook Time: 25 minutes

4 Servings

INGREDIENTS

1 ½ cups flour

1 tsp cinnamon

3 eggs

2 tsp baking powder

½ tsp sugar

1 cup milk

2 tbsp butter, melted

1 tbsp yogurt

1 zucchini, shredded

A pinch of salt

2 tbsp cream cheese

DIRECTIONS

Preheat air fryer to 350 F.

In a bowl, whisk the eggs with sugar, salt, cinnamon, cream cheese, flour, and baking powder.

In another bowl, combine the remaining ingredients, except for the zucchini.

Gently combine the dry and liquid mixtures.

Stir in zucchini.

Grease the muffin tins with cooking spray and pour the batter inside them.

Place in the air fryer and cook for 18 minutes.

Serve warm or chilled.

Banana & Hazelnut Muffins

Prep + Cook Time: 30 minutes

6 Servings

INGREDIENTS

¼ cup butter, melted

¼ cup honey

1 egg, lightly beaten

2 ripe bananas, mashed

½ tsp vanilla extract

1 cup flour

½ tsp baking powder

½ tsp ground cinnamon

¼ cup hazelnuts, chopped

¼ cup dark chocolate chips

DIRECTIONS

Spray a muffin tin that fits in your air fryer with cooking spray.

In a bowl, whisk butter, honey, eggs, bananas, and vanilla until well combined.

Sift in flour, baking powder, and cinnamon without overmixing. Stir in the hazelnuts and chocolate.

Pour the batter into the muffin holes and fit in the air fryer.

Cook for 20 minutes at 350 F on Bake, checking them around the 15-minute mark.

Serve chilled.

Breakfast Banana Bread

Prep + Cook Time: 30 minutes

2 Servings

INGREDIENTS

1 cup flour

¼ tsp baking soda 1

 tsp baking powder

⅓ cup sugar

2 mashed bananas

¼ cup vegetable oil

1 egg, beaten

1 tsp vanilla extract

¾ cup chopped walnuts

¼ tsp salt

2 tbsp peanut butter, softened

2 tbsp sour cream

DIRECTIONS

Preheat air fryer to 350 F.

Sift the flour into a large bowl and add salt, baking powder, and baking soda; stir to combine.

In another bowl, combine the bananas, vegetable oil, egg, peanut butter, vanilla, sugar, and sour cream; stir.

Mix both mixtures and fold in the chopped walnuts.

Pour the batter into a greased baking dish and fit in the fryer.

Bake for 20-25 minutes until nice and golden.

Serve chilled.

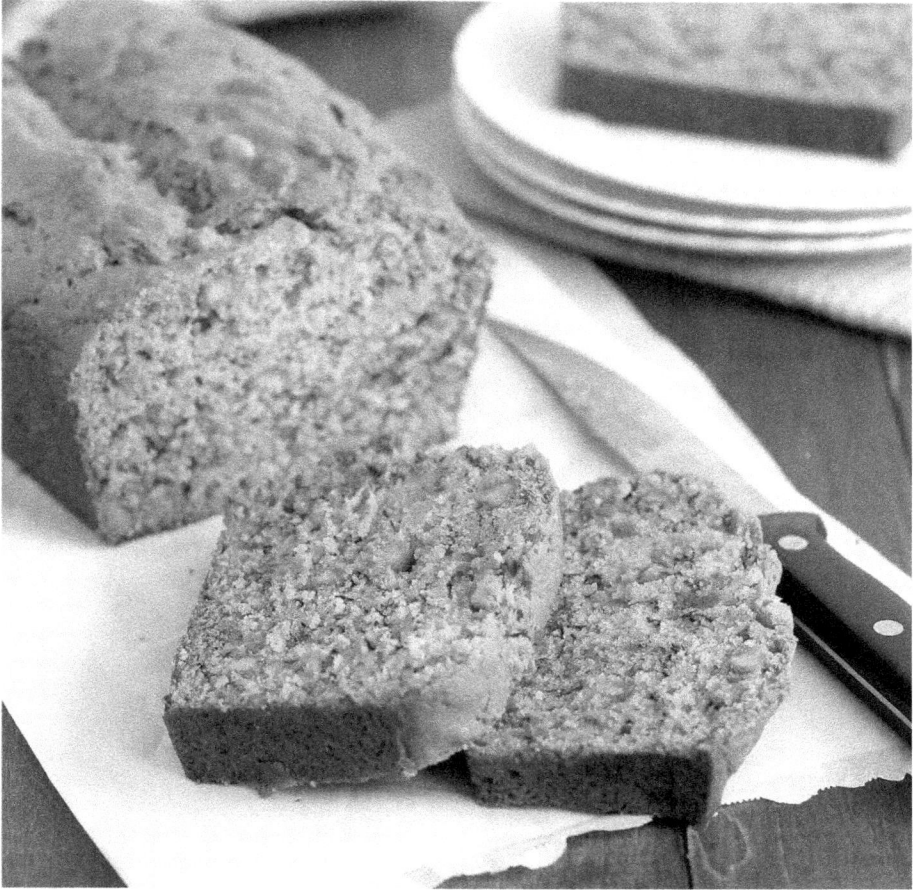

Sweet Bread Pudding with Raisins

Prep + Cook Time: 45 minutes

4 Servings

INGREDIENTS

8 bread slices, cubed

½ cup buttermilk

¼ cup honey

1 cup milk

2 eggs

½ tsp vanilla extract

2 tbsp butter, softened

¼ cup sugar

4 tbsp raisins

2 tbsp chopped hazelnuts

Ground cinnamon for garnish

DIRECTIONS

Preheat air fryer to 350 F.

Beat the eggs with buttermilk, honey, milk, vanilla, sugar, and butter in a bowl.

Stir in raisins and hazelnuts, then add in the bread cubes to soak, about 10 minutes.

Transfer to a greased tin and Bake the pudding in fryer for 25 minutes.

Dust with ground cinnamon and serve.

Cherry & Almond Scones

Prep + Cook Time: 25 minutes

4 Servings

INGREDIENTS

2 cups flour + some more

⅓ cup sugar

2 tsp baking powder

½ cup sliced almonds

¾ cup chopped cherries, dried

¼ cup cold butter, cut into cubes

½ cup milk

1 egg

1 tsp vanilla extract

DIRECTIONS

Line the air fryer basket with baking paper.

Mix together flour, sugar, baking powder, sliced almonds, and dried cherries in a bowl.

Rub the butter into the dry ingredients with hands to form a sandy, crumbly texture.

Whisk together egg, milk, and vanilla extract.

Pour into the dry ingredients and stir to combine.

Sprinkle a working board with flour, lay the dough onto the board, and give it a few kneads.

Shape into a rectangle and cut into 9 squares.

Arrange the squares in the air fryer's basket and cook for 14 minutes at 390 F.

Work in batches if needed.

Serve immediately.

Toasted Herb & Garlic Bagel

Prep + Cook Time: 10 minutes

1 Serving

INGREDIENTS

1 tbsp butter, softened

¼ tsp dried basil

¼ tsp dried parsley

¼ tsp garlic powder

1 tbsp Parmesan cheese, grated

Salt and black pepper to taste

1 bagel, halved

DIRECTIONS

Preheat air fryer to 370 degrees.

Place the bagel halves in the fryer and toast for 3 minutes on AirFry mode.

Mix butter, Parmesan cheese, garlic, basil, and parsley in a bowl.

Season with salt and pepper.

Spread the mixture onto the toasted bagel and return to the fryer to AirFry for 3 more minutes.

Serve.

Spanish Chorizo Frittata

Prep + Cook Time: 20 minutes

2 Servings

INGREDIENTS

4 eggs

1 large potato, boiled and cubed

½ cup sweet corn

½ cup feta cheese, crumbled

1 tbsp parsley, chopped

1 chorizo sausage, sliced

2 tbsp olive oil

Salt and black pepper to taste

DIRECTIONS

Preheat air fryer to 330 F.

Heat olive oil in a skillet over medium heat and cook the chorizo until slightly browned, about 4 minutes; set aside.

In a bowl, beat the eggs with salt and black pepper.

Stir in all of the remaining ingredients, except for the parsley.

Grease a baking pan that fits your air fryer with the chorizo fat and pour in the egg mixture.

Insert into the air fryer and Bake for 8-10 minutes until golden.

Serve topped with parsley.

Enjoy!

Easy Breakfast Potatoes

Prep + Cook Time: 35 minutes

6 Servings

INGREDIENTS

4 large potatoes, cubed

2 bell peppers, cut into 1-inch chunks

½ onion, diced

2 tsp olive oil

1 garlic clove, minced

½ tsp dried thyme

½ tsp cayenne pepper

Salt to taste

DIRECTIONS

Preheat air fryer to 390 F.

Place the potato cubes in a bowl and sprinkle with garlic, cayenne pepper, and salt.

Drizzle with some olive oil and toss to coat.

Arrange the potatoes on an even layer on the greased air fryer basket.

Air Fry for 10 minutes, shaking the basket once during the cooking time.

In the meantime, add the remaining olive oil, garlic, thyme, and salt in a mixing bowl.

Add in the bell peppers and onion and mix well.

Pour the veggies over the potatoes and continue cooking in the air fryer for 5 minutes.

At the 5-minute mark, shake the basket and cook for 5 minutes.

Serve warm.

Air Fried Shirred Eggs

Prep + Cook Time: 20 minutes

2 Servings

INGREDIENTS

2 tsp butter

4 eggs

2 tbsp heavy cream

4 slices ham

3 tbsp Parmesan cheese, grated

¼ tsp paprika

Salt and black pepper to taste

2 tsp chopped chives

DIRECTIONS

Preheat air fryer to 320 F.

Arrange the ham slices on the bottom of a greased pie pan to cover it completely.

Whisk one egg along with the heavy cream, salt, and pepper in a small bowl.

Pour the mixture over the ham slices.

Crack the other eggs on top and sprinkle with Parmesan cheese.

AirFry for 14 minutes.

Garnish with paprika and fresh chives and serve.

Pancake The German Way

Prep + Cook Time: 30 minutes

4 Servings

INGREDIENTS

3 eggs, beaten

2 tbsp butter, melted

1 cup flour

2 tbsp sugar, powdered

½ cup milk

1 cup fresh strawberries, sliced

DIRECTIONS

Preheat air fryer to 330 F.

In a bowl, mix flour, milk, and eggs until fully incorporated.

Grease a baking pan that fits in your air fryer with the butter and pour in the mixture.

Place the pan in the air fryer's basket and AirFry for 12-16 minutes until the pancake is fluffy and golden brown.

Drizzle powdered sugar and arrange sliced strawberries on top to serve.

Masala Omelet the Indian Way

Prep + Cook Time: 15 minutes

1 Serving

INGREDIENTS

1 garlic clove, crushed

2 green onions

½ chili powder

½ tsp garam masala

2 eggs

1 tbsp olive oil 1

 tbsp fresh cilantro, chopped

Salt and black pepper to taste

DIRECTIONS

Warm the olive oil in a skillet over medium.

Add and sauté the spring onions and garlic for 2 minutes until softened.

Sprinkle with chili powder, garam masala, salt, and pepper.

Set aside.

Preheat air fryer to 340 F.

In a bowl, mix the eggs with salt and black pepper.

Add in the masala mixture and stir well.

Transfer to a greased baking that fits into your air fryer.

Bake in the fryer for 8 minutes until golden, flipping once.

Scatter your omelet with cilantro and serve immediately.

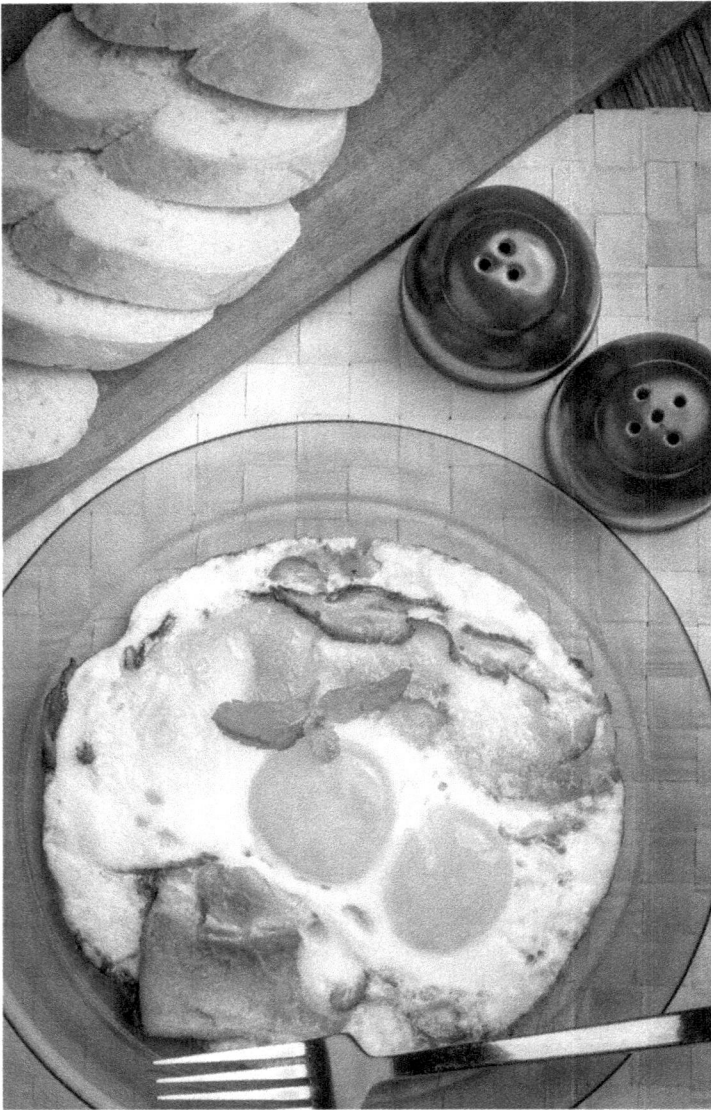

www.ingramcontent.com/pod-product-compliance
Lightning Source LLC
Chambersburg PA
CBHW070721030426
42336CB00013B/1885